Faith Hill
Gay Gray

WHAT IS
HEALTH?

Oxford University Press

Oxford University Press, Walton Street, Oxford OX2 6DP

Oxford   New York   Toronto
Delhi   Bombay   Calcutta   Madras   Karachi
Petaling Jaya   Singapore   Hong Kong   Tokyo
Nairobi   Dar es Salaam   Cape Town
Melbourne   Auckland

and associated companies in
Berlin   Ibadan

Oxford is a trade mark of Oxford University Press

© Faith Hill and Gay Gray 1990

ISBN 0 19 832622 X

Phototypeset in Univers and Century Old Style by
Tradespools Limited, Frome, Somerset

Printed by Ebenezer Baylis Limited, Worcester

Acknowledgements

The illustrations are by: **Peter Ahern, Susan
Beresford, Ed Carr, Nick Duffy, Jean Hands,
Beverly Levy, Chris Price** and **Mike Sharp**.

The photos were provided by: **BUGA UP** 14; **Cull
Photographic** 5; **Format/Maggie Murray** 3; /**Brenda
Prince** 4; **Sally and Richard Greenhill** 8; **Network/
Barry Lewis** 26 (right), /**Martin Mayer** 26 (left).

The book cover on page 29 is reproduced by permission of
Longman Group UK Ltd.

CONTENTS

What Does 'Being Healthy' Mean to You?   2

Looking Back in Time   6

Global Thinking   8

Health as a Triangle   10

The Health Bandwagon   12

Unhealthy Adverts   14

Making Sense of it All   16

Can we be Healthy all the Time?   18

Choices   19

Is it Easy to be Healthy?   20

Freedom of Choice   22

Health For All   24

The National Health Service   26

Support Groups   28

»

What Does 'Being Healthy' Mean to You?

People's idea of 'health' will vary depending, to a great extent, on the country and times in which they live and on what is going on around them. So for you, living in Britain at the present time, what does 'being healthy' mean? The following quiz might help you to find out.

Looking at the list below tick the statements which you agree with. Tick as many as you like.

For me, being healthy means:

1 Being able to run a mile. ☐

2 Never getting anything more serious than a slight cold or upset stomach. ☐

3 Being able to get on well with people. ☐

4 Avoiding taking/eating/doing things which might shorten my life, e.g. smoking and hard drugs. ☐

5 Having a good figure. ☐

6 Being able to touch my toes. ☐

7 Having ways of coping with unwanted stress. ☐

8 Caring about other people. ☐

9 Having a regular exercise routine, e.g. playing a sport, doing aerobics or weight-training. ☐

10 Hardly ever going to the doctor. ☐

11 Feeling that deep down, I'm OK. ☐

12 Avoiding anything that might make me ill or give me an infection. ☐

13 Being able to adapt and make the best of the situation I'm in. ☐

14 Not having spots or pimples. ☐

15 Living to be 80 years old ☐

16 Being able to cope with changes in life, e.g. leaving home or college, unemployment or a new job. ☐

If possible, before you check your answers, compare them with those of a friend. Are there many differences or are most of your answers the same? Remember every individual is likely to hold different views on what it means to be healthy.

Now compare your answers with the comments given on the following pages.

Healthy is . . . being fit

If you have ticked against statements 1, 6 and 9, then you probably think of being healthy in terms of physical fitness. Mental and physical health can be closely linked. Have you ever found yourself caught in the vicious circle of not feeling good about yourself or your life, so that you stop looking after yourself and stop worrying about whether you are fit or not . . . which in turn leads to you not feeling fit or good about yourself. . . .

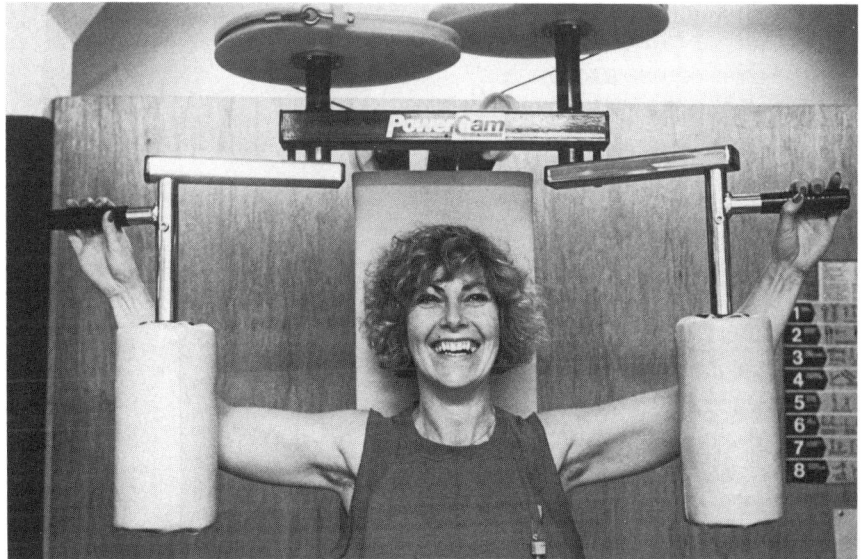

But you can be physically fit and still be unhealthy. *Or* you may not be able to run a mile, but you might still feel healthy. Disabled people have shown time and time again that they can lead healthy lives, in spite of their disabilities.

Healthy is . . . living a long time

Ticking against statements 4 and 15 suggests that, for you, being healthy means living to an old age. The health of the nation is frequently measured by how long people live. We try to identify factors which may affect our chances of living a long, healthy life. Such factors would include:

● What we eat and drink.
● Whether we are employed or not.
● If we have a job, what working conditions we have.
● Where we live (what sort of housing conditions?)
● Whether we smoke.

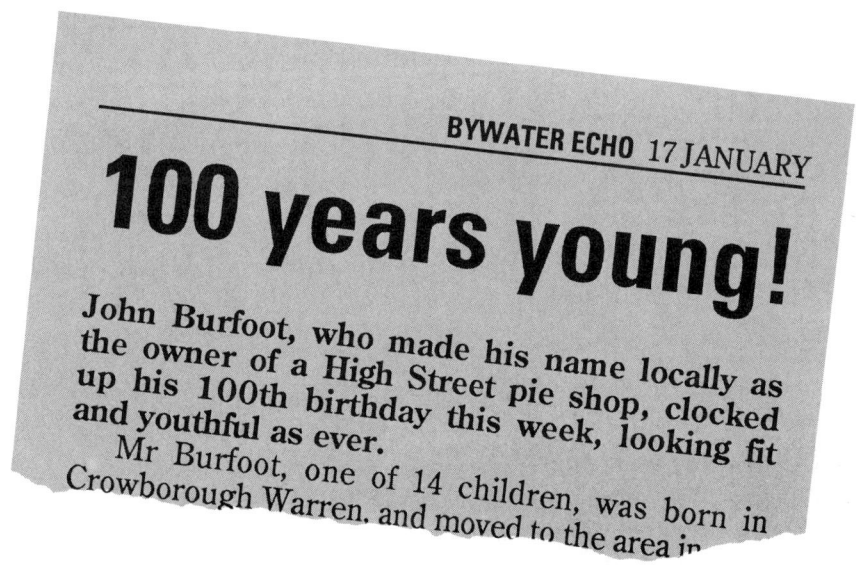

BYWATER ECHO 17 JANUARY

100 years young!

John Burfoot, who made his name locally as the owner of a High Street pie shop, clocked up his 100th birthday this week, looking fit and youthful as ever.

Mr Burfoot, one of 14 children, was born in Crowborough Warren, and moved to the area in

But is living to 100 what *you* are aiming for? Some people live to a ripe old age, but no longer really enjoy life. Some find that in retirement they have the freedom to enjoy life that they've never had before. Living to an old age is one measure of health, but on its own it does not necessarily mean a person is healthy.

Healthy is . . . adapting

If you have ticked against statements 7, 13 and 16, you probably think of health as the ability to adapt to whatever situation you find yourself in. It can be argued that nowadays the world is changing at a rapid pace – work patterns, values, the way we live, the roles of men and women are all being challenged. A person needs to be able to cope with all these changes in order to adapt.

Often people look for an easy answer to help them through difficult patches. Some take anti-depressants (Valium is still the most prescribed drug in the world). Some take to drinking alcohol to drown their sorrows and help them cope. Certain ways of coping with change are definitely less healthy than others!

Family Announcements

BIRTHS, MARRIAGES and DEATHS

Broken marriage led to suicide

A nurse took her own life because she was unhappy at her marriage breaking up after 17 years.
Mrs P

Teenagers joining the dole queues

THE number of youngsters on the dole in the country has increased by 50 per cent, new figures revealed today.
Last month 2,305 young people were on the official books and available on the job market.
That is despite

Trauma of axed jobs

Healthy is . . . not being ill

Ticking against statements 2, 10 and 12 suggests that health for you means avoiding illness. Many people only start to think about their health once they are ill. It is then that we turn to doctors and the National Health Service to help us to put things right . . . and then that we start to be concerned if the service is not adequate!

But is 'not being ill' a measure of 'health'?

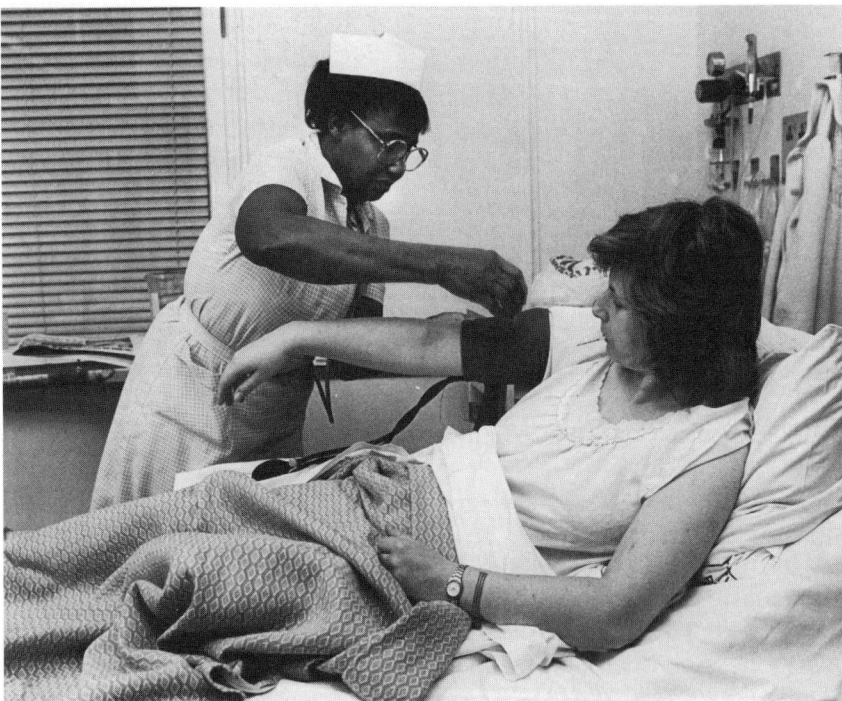

Healthy is . . . looking good

If you ticked against statements 5 or 14, you probably think health has something to do with your appearance. Health products are big business. Manufacturers spend a fortune trying to persuade us to buy their goods, with phrases like 'What girl doesn't want beautiful legs?' and 'If you have tried everything and still have spots, blemishes, blackheads, dry skin; write to us and we'll show you how to have that clear complexion you've always wanted'. Do you know anyone who is completely happy with how they look? Most people would like to be either thinner or taller, more feminine or 'macho' or to have a different nose, or feet, or breasts, or legs . . . the list is endless!

But what has all this to do with health? Doubtless there is a connection in that your skin condition or weight can be a reflection of your state of health; if you look good, you often feel good. But worrying too much about your appearance could be very unhealthy! There are some things about ourselves that we can't, and don't need to change.

Healthy is . . . feeling good, getting on with others

Ticking against numbers 3, 8 and 11, shows that you probably think of health in connection with feeling good and getting on well with people. You could say that this is looking at health in a positive way. It is more difficult to measure than illness and physical health. It covers how we feel about ourselves and others – our emotional and social health. Can we say we are really healthy if we don't take these things into account?

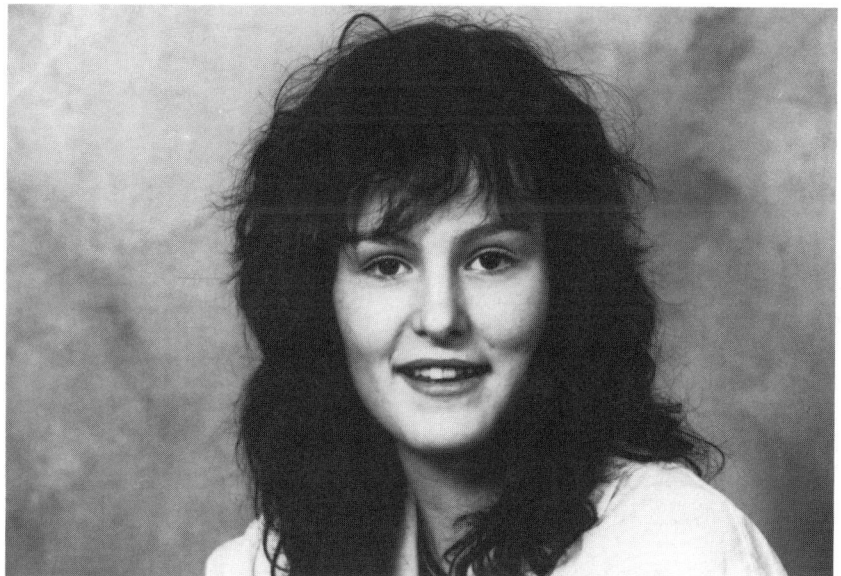

Well . . . what do you think?

Perhaps you ticked against statements from all these groups. As health is a mixture of all the things mentioned, this would hardly be surprising.

Now compare your responses to the quiz with the others in your group. Did you tick different numbers to your friends? Different responses are also to be expected. The important thing is to work out what being healthy means to you . . . and what it might take to achieve it.

Looking Back in Time

People's views of health depend partly on the times in which they live. If survival is constantly threatened by disease and famine, health may be seen in purely physical terms. It is then defined as the absence of illness and early death.

If we look back in history we can see that there were times when people had trouble just staying alive. For example, in the Fourteenth Century in England, a series of epidemics wiped out half the population between 1348 and 1375. Some small villages were killed off completely.

The main cause of this was a bacterium which led to 'the plague'. This was accompanied by widespread outbreaks of smallpox, typhus and dysentery. It is hard to imagine what it must have been like to live in a time when so many people were ill and dying.

Of course, Britain's history hasn't all been as gloomy as the time of the plague. But it wasn't until the 1850s – only just over a hundred years ago – that the threat of infectious diseases began to disappear.

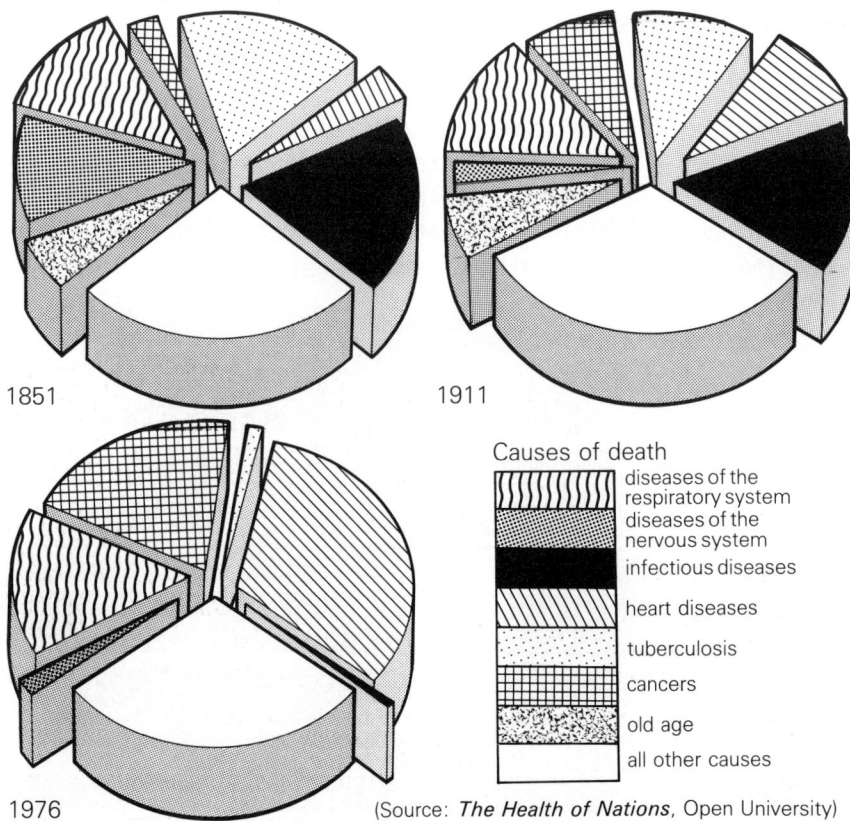

1851

1911

1976

Causes of death

	diseases of the respiratory system
	diseases of the nervous system
	infectious diseases
	heart diseases
	tuberculosis
	cancers
	old age
	all other causes

(Source: *The Health of Nations*, Open University)

Experts disagree as to why the improvements occurred, and deaths due to infectious diseases declined, but there appears to be a mixture of reasons. These include:

● Medical intervention – immunization, antibiotics, etc.
● Improved sanitation – clean water supply, sewers.
● Better nutrition and a better standard of living – increasing people's resistance to illness.

As all of these factors contributed to the high standard of health we now enjoy, it is easy to see why many people think that 'health' is *just* about keeping clean, eating properly and going to the doctor regularly.

» During the worst outbreaks of the plague nearly half the population died in 25 years. What do you think our attitudes to health would be if we were faced with a similar problem today? What would we worry about most and how would we change our way of life?

» We are still a long way from curing all infectious diseases and AIDS is now becoming a real threat to health. How do you think AIDS should *best* be tackled:

● More information made available, so that people can change their life-style?
● More money spent on research to find a cure?
● Isolate all people who are HIV positive?
● Some other way.

In order to consider the issues involved, you could discuss the points in a small group. Or you could 'role-play' a debate, each taking up one point of view that is not necessarily your own.

» You could find out more about infectious diseases and their decline by interviewing some elderly people in your neighbourhood. Some points you could raise with them include:

> What do they remember about the causes of illness when they were young?

> Why do they think these illnesses have declined?

> What were the main things they were taught about health when they were young?

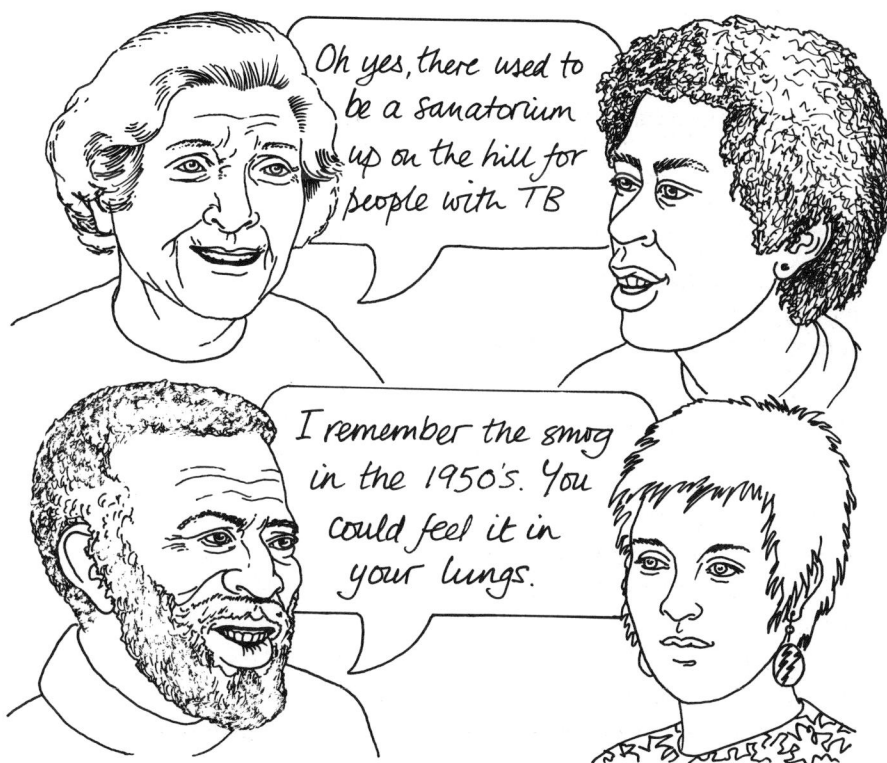

Oh yes, there used to be a sanatorium up on the hill for people with TB

I remember the smog in the 1950's. You could feel it in your lungs.

If your local community includes people born in other parts of the world, you could compare their memories with those of people you have interviewed who were born in Britain.

Global Thinking

Just as history will affect views on health, so will geography. Where people live is bound to have an effect on their outlook on life.

Most people in 'rich' countries like our own *expect* to be fairly healthy. And often if they feel something is wrong with their health, they expect their doctor to find out what it is and to do something about it.

The situation is very different in most third world countries. There people may live a long way from a doctor and are used to putting up with painful and life-threatening conditions, which we might find it hard to tolerate. Malnutrition and other problems which affect health are often accepted as nothing out of the ordinary.

However, many of the diseases common in third world countries could be prevented. Clean water supplies and good food can rapidly build up resistance to disease, and immunization can prevent the spread of infections. So, people in these countries *do* have a right to expect a higher level of health.

In the richer countries, many of us contribute to our own poor health and our diseases are often difficult to cure. Some of the most common, such as heart disease and cancer, are clearly linked to our way of life. Some of us smoke, drink vast quantities of alcohol, eat all the wrong things, never take any exercise, and drive around as if our bodies were resistant to any impact.

The way some of us treat our bodies is a bit like running a car: when it goes wrong you can always take it to the garage to have it fixed!

But these attitudes and patterns of behaviour may also be linked to *where* we live. The speed of life causes emotional stress and living in our society has its own problems and difficulties.

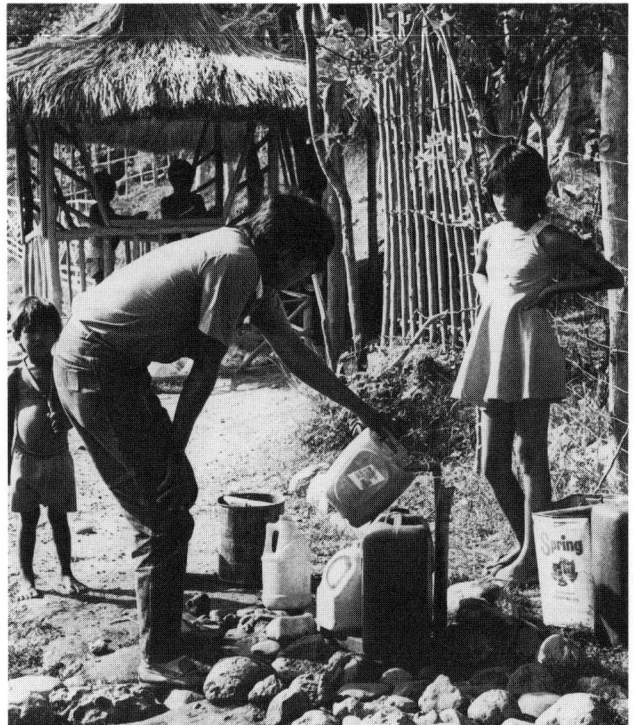

ACTIVITIES

» Do you think it's true that people view being healthy in a similar way to a car that goes well? Think about or discuss the advantages and the disadvantages of this view of health.

» If you have time for a longer project, two groups could research and prepare two separate displays. One could cover health and illness in Britain today. The other could cover the same points for developing countries. The two displays could then be mounted and could lead to discussions about the differences and similarities concerning global aspects of health.

The material in the chart opposite, may help you to decide which information to include in your display.

In the rich countries of the North

Diseases of affluence
Cancers and cardiovascular disease are the two main causes of death. These are often caused by the environment and by personal lifestyles, such as smoking and the food we eat.

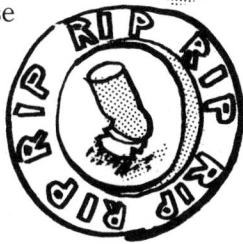

Mental illness
The North spends a fortune on tranquillizers and other drugs for stress and mental illness. Over a million Europeans are in mental homes.

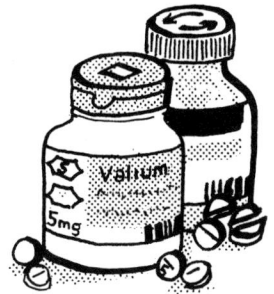

Increasing numbers of elderly
The percentage of elderly people is increasing rapidly in the North. They often suffer from isolation as well as ill-health.

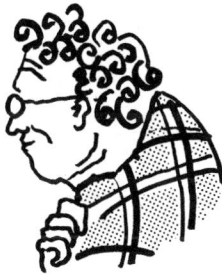

High tech medicine
Much of the health budget is spent on expensive hospital treatment and amazing surgery such as heart/lung transplants. But some people think that more of this money should be spent on preventing diseases.

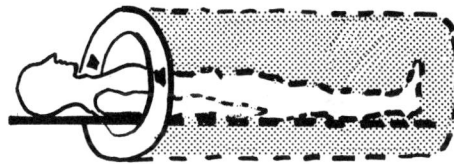

In the Third World

Child health
The biggest problem in the Third World is the number of deaths amongst babies and small children. In some countries infant mortality is as high as 210 out of every 1,000 infants. (Compared with an average of 19 in the North)

Main causes of infant deaths:
Diarrhoea, Malnutrition and Infectious diseases.

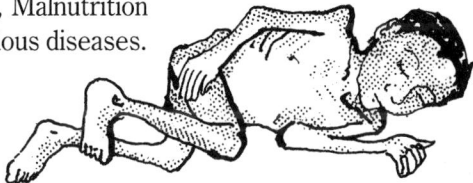

Waterborne diseases
Several hundred million people suffer from diseases spread by dirty water. This includes diseases such as typhoid, cholera, dysentery and diarrhoea.

Water-breeding insects, such as mosquitoes, carry malaria and yellow fever. River blindness and other diseases are spread by worms and larvae entering the body from water.

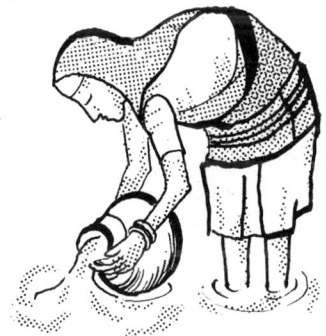

Health care
Although there is so much need in the Third World, much less is spent on health than in the North. Sometimes expensive hospitals are built in the towns, far from needy people in the countryside.

In the North, there are over 50 medical personnel per 10,000 people. In many parts of the Third World, there are less than 10 personnel per 10,000 people.

Immunization
Only 20 per cent of the world's children are protected against measles, whooping cough, polio, T.B., tetanus and diphtheria. These are major killers in the Third World.

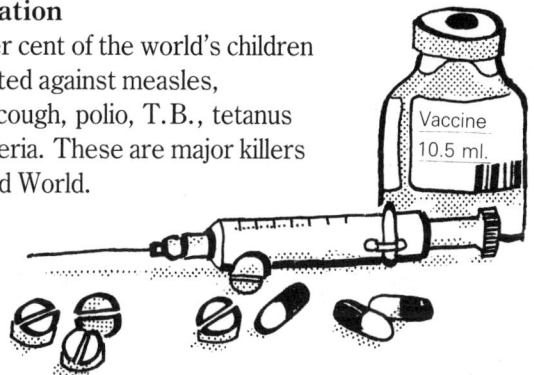

Further information

The statistics given here are from *The Gaia Atlas of Planet Management.*
Ed. Norman Myers. Another useful resource is *The Health of Nations*
produced by the Open University.

Health as a Triangle

Another way of viewing health is to see it as a triangle. This idea is based on the thinking of an American called Abraham Maslow. He put forward a theory that all our needs are built one upon another, with the most fundamental forming the base of a triangle.

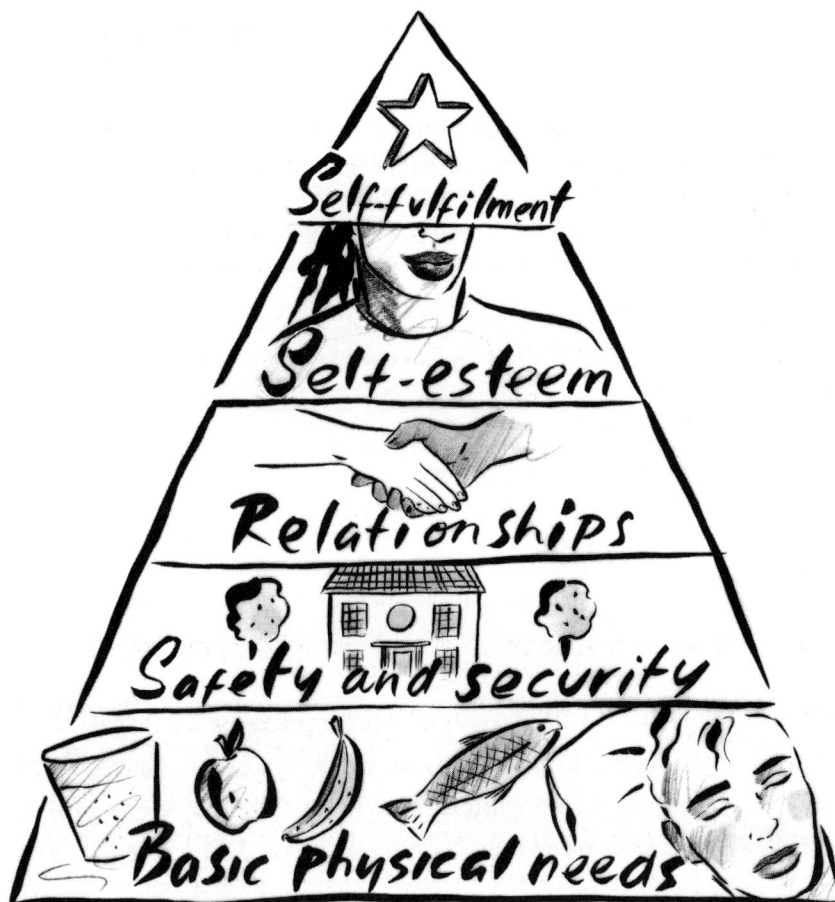

At the bottom we have needs such as water, food and sleep. Without this level we cannot survive. Next, we need to feel safe from personal or environmental danger.

Having satisfied these essential needs, the triangle becomes more complicated. We also need supporting, caring relationships and the sense of belonging to a group. This means having a family and friends. Then we need to be sure of our own personal worth: our self-esteem. This means we have to recognize the importance of self-respect and personal approval of ourselves; i.e. liking ourselves.

At the very top of the triangle, Maslow included the idea of self-fulfilment. This means that each person has to strive for a goal that they feel is important for their life. It's about there being a sense of direction, a purpose to reach out for, in everybody's life. For some people, this may involve a religious commitment or belief in a particular religious teaching, for example, Christianity or Islam. But for other people, self-fulfilment may mean following a different path. They may strive to be a pop star or football hero. People commit themselves to many different causes and strive for different goals in life.

Health may be seen as the *whole* triangle. The different parts are all important and all go together to make up a healthy person.

» Draw a large triangle on paper and divide it into Maslow's five sections. For each section, write in as many examples as you can think of that relate to that particular need. For example, in the bottom section include 'food' and 'water'. Then think about or discuss some of the following points:

● How easy/difficult is it to think of needs for each section?
● Are some of the needs more important to health than others?
● Can you be healthy if one of the sections is permanently missing from your life?
● Is it possible to meet all the needs, all of the time?
● Do you feel that you would like to meet certain needs that you are not fulfilling at the moment? If so, could you change your situation to achieve this? How?
● Could it ever be 'selfish' to view your own health in this way?
● Overall, do you think this is a useful way of viewing health?

» Maslow writes a lot about self-fulfilment and the importance of a purpose in life. You may find it useful to brainstorm some of the many different goals people have in their lives and to think about where you fit into all this. For example:

● Do you have a purpose in life?
● Do you need a purpose in order to be 'healthy'?
● Do you want a purpose?

Example brainstorm: yours may look completely different!

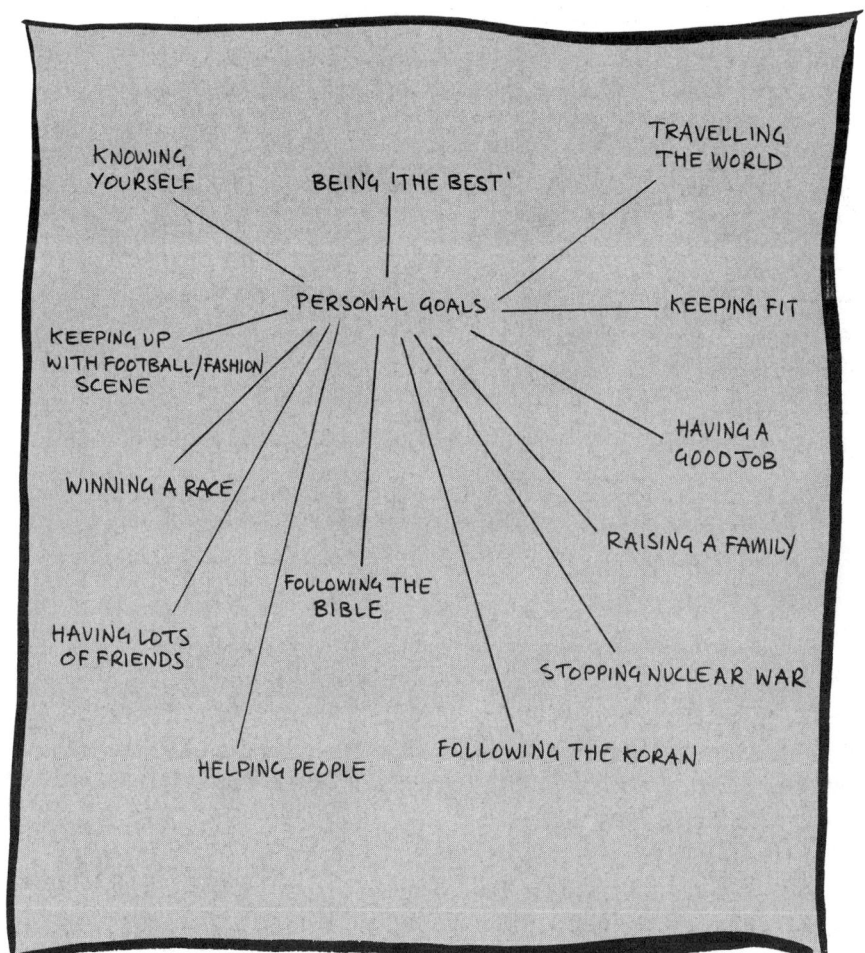

KNOWING YOURSELF · BEING 'THE BEST' · TRAVELLING THE WORLD · KEEPING UP WITH FOOTBALL/FASHION SCENE · PERSONAL GOALS · KEEPING FIT · HAVING A GOOD JOB · WINNING A RACE · RAISING A FAMILY · FOLLOWING THE BIBLE · HAVING LOTS OF FRIENDS · STOPPING NUCLEAR WAR · HELPING PEOPLE · FOLLOWING THE KORAN

The Health Bandwagon

Every day we are bombarded with messages about health – in the newspapers, in magazines, on the television – it's difficult to get away from it!

On this page you will find a selection of health messages, introduced through advertising during the 1980s. Can you identify the agency, manufacturer or organization which was responsible for these messages? The answers are given upside down at the bottom of the page.

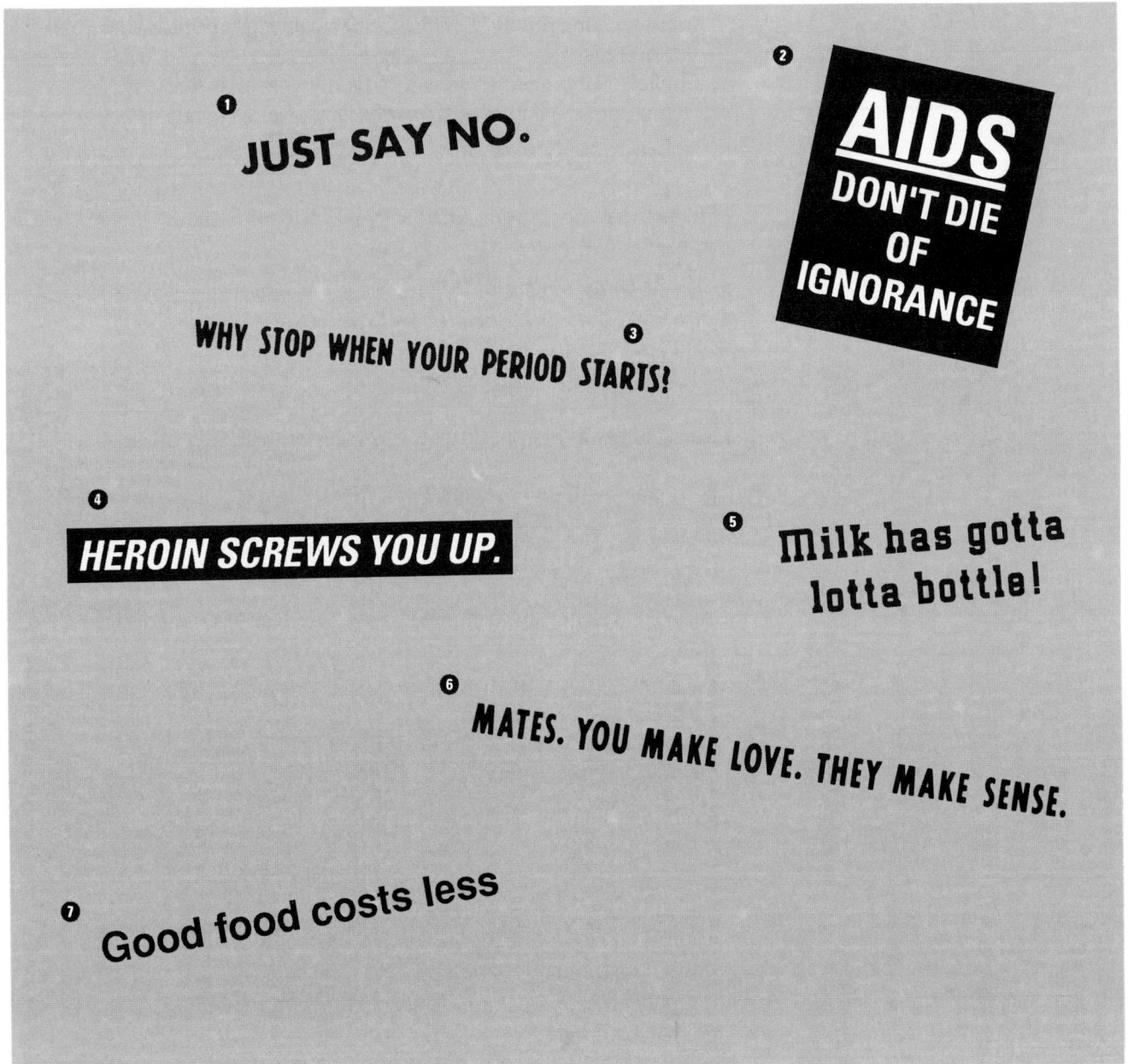

❶ JUST SAY NO.

❷ **AIDS** DON'T DIE OF IGNORANCE

❸ WHY STOP WHEN YOUR PERIOD STARTS!

❹ **HEROIN SCREWS YOU UP.**

❺ Milk has gotta lotta bottle!

❻ MATES. YOU MAKE LOVE. THEY MAKE SENSE.

❼ Good food costs less

Since the time that this booklet was written, there are likely to have been other campaigns, adverts or messages about health. Can you think of any?

» Pair up with someone else. You have 5 minutes to list as many 'health messages' from recent campaigns or adverts as you can. Make sure you know who was responsible for them and list their names separately.

Give your messages to another pair. Can they identify the source? Who gave the message?

Compare the results. Had you listed many of the same ones? Which campaigns or adverts seem to have had some impact? If slogans are remembered, does this necessarily influence the way in which people behave?

» With two or three other people, look through a number of magazines and newspapers, cutting out any articles or advertisements which have something to do with health.

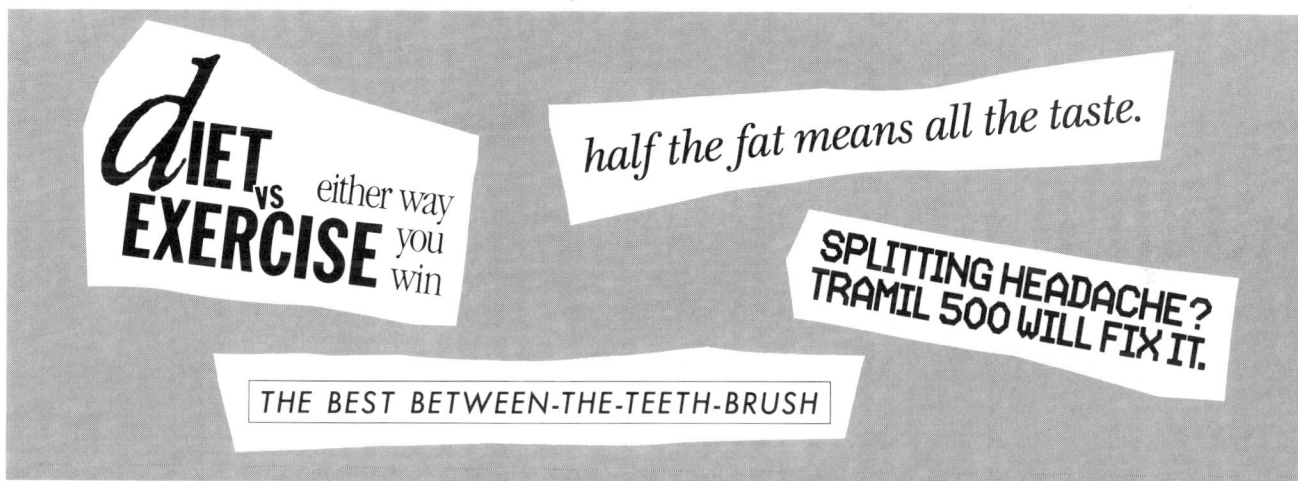

DIET vs EXERCISE *either way you win*

half the fat means all the taste.

SPLITTING HEADACHE? TRAMIL 500 WILL FIX IT.

THE BEST BETWEEN-THE-TEETH-BRUSH

Which publications contain the largest number of references to health? Why might this be so?

Can you group the cuttings in any way? You might decide that you have quite a few:

● On a particular health issue, such as keeping fit or AIDS;
● Which are aimed at women;
● Which are out to sell a certain product.

Choose one group of health cuttings to display for others to see, e.g. by making a collage on a large sheet of paper.

Compare your display with other people's. Discuss the number of health messages which you have noticed in various publications.

Some reasons for writing about health:

● To sell a certain product.
● It's 'News', e.g. the results of recent research.
● To encourage people to lead a healthy life.
● It's a current health issue which is of general interest.

Can you identify any others?

Health is a major issue and big business.

In 1987/8 direct government spending on alcohol misuse was £553,756.

Each year the Government receives around £6 billion revenue from taxes on alcohol.

Unhealthy Adverts

One of the biggest debates of our times is about whether companies should be allowed to advertise unhealthy products. People feel strongly about any restrictions on freedom and, anyway, who's to say what is an unhealthy product? After all, even the most innocent products can be harmful sometimes.

But in some cases we have very good reasons to be sure that even a small amount of a product is bad for people – like cigarettes. Yet we still go on advertising cigarettes and at the same time include a Government Health Warning. Does this make any sense?

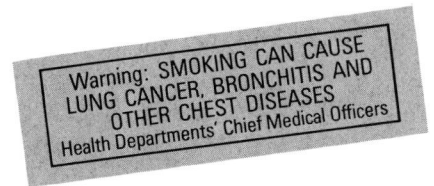

Warning: SMOKING CAN CAUSE LUNG CANCER, BRONCHITIS AND OTHER CHEST DISEASES
Health Departments' Chief Medical Officers

Some groups, including doctors and medical students, think not. They say we should ban all smoking adverts straightaway.

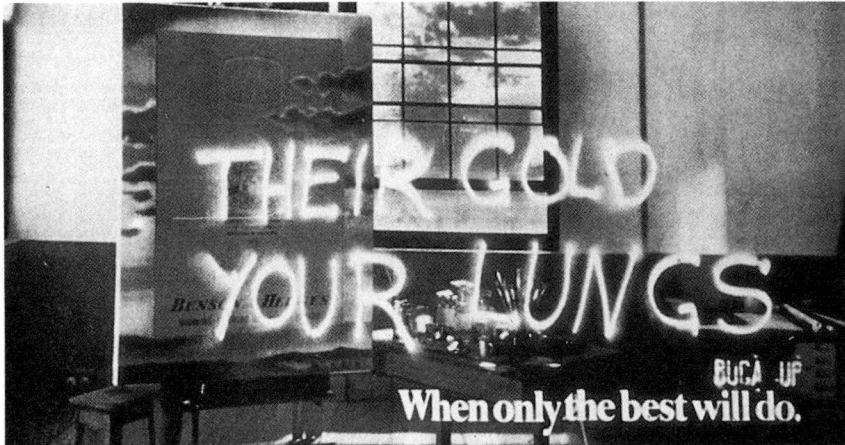

THEIR GOLD YOUR LUNGS
BUGA UP
When only the best will do.

In Australia, there are many doctors, health workers and others who are so determined to stop the advertising of cigarettes that they have formed into a group called BUGA-UP. This stands for 'Billboard Utilizing Graffitists Against Unhealthy Promotions': in plain English, changing adverts with spray-cans of paint!

What BUGA-UP is doing is, of course, *illegal* both here and in Australia. But they believe it's the only way of stopping the tobacco companies.

There are groups involved in similar protests in England, including:

TREES,
P.O. Box 316,
LONDON   E2 9PP

AGHAST,
93 Cromwell Road,
BRISTOL   BS6 5EX

NO ADS

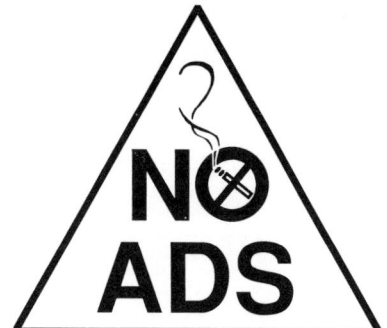

Did you know that every year the tobacco industry spends over £100 million on advertising its products? Three of the world's six largest tobacco companies are based in Britain: Imperial Tobacco, Rothmans International and British American Tobacco (BAT).

Is graffiti ever justified. What do you think?

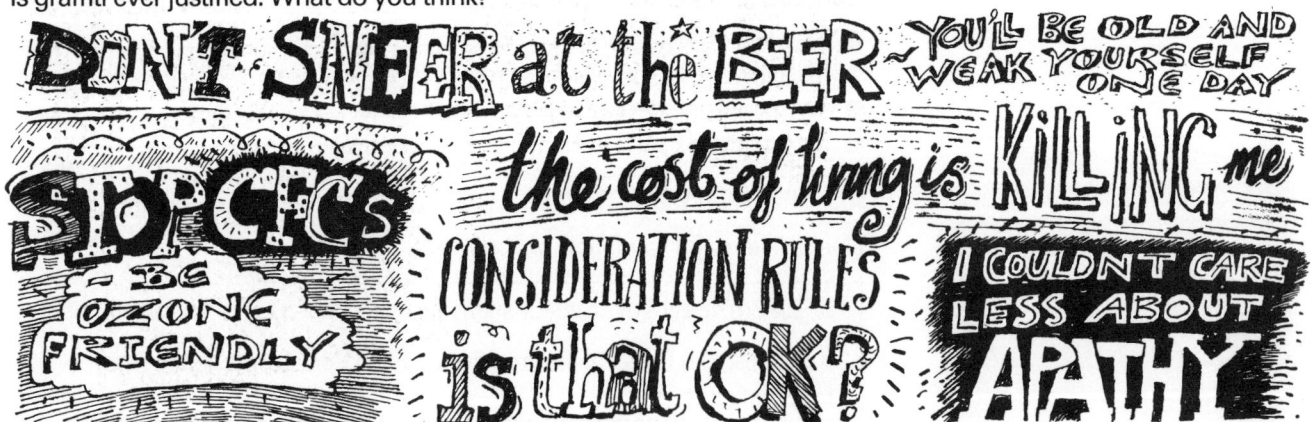

DON'T SNEER at the BEER ~ YOU'LL BE OLD AND WEAK YOURSELF ONE DAY

STOP CFCs ~ BE OZONE FRIENDLY

the cost of living is KILLING me

CONSIDERATION RULES is that OK?

I COULDN'T CARE LESS ABOUT APATHY

» Cut out magazine adverts for cigarettes and have a go at your own BUGA-UP with felt pens.

» Contact TREES and AGHAST for more information about what they do.

» Keep a record of the number of adverts which you see for cigarettes during the next week. Where did you see them? What form did they take, e.g. on billboards or in magazines?

There are some restrictions on the way in which cigarettes can be advertised, including the following:

No cigarette adverts on TV since 1965.

A Government Health Warning to be added to cigarette adverts (since 1986 there are alternative warnings).

No promotion or advert should have special appeal to young people, e.g. no popular celebrity can be used; it must not appear 'macho' to smoke.

How do cigarette manufacturers get round this?

» Research in Manchester in 1984 showed that when questioned about which cigarette brands they were familiar with, young people replied with the names of brands which had recently been on the TV through hours of sponsored sporting events, such as snooker. Find out more about the extent of sponsorship by cigarette companies and the restrictions imposed at present.

» If you want more information about advertising regulations, you could contact the Advertising Standards Authority and ask for an abridged copy of the Advertising Code.

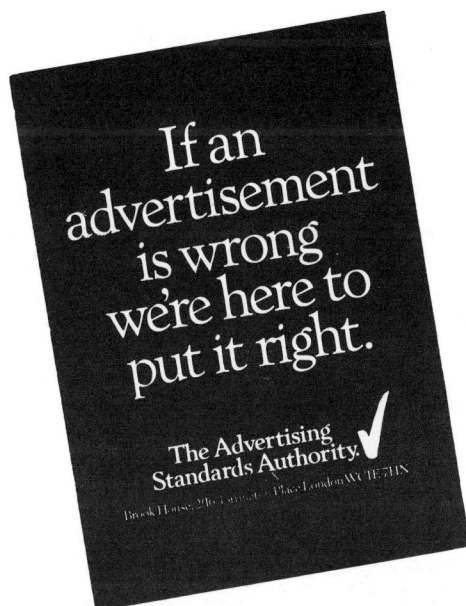

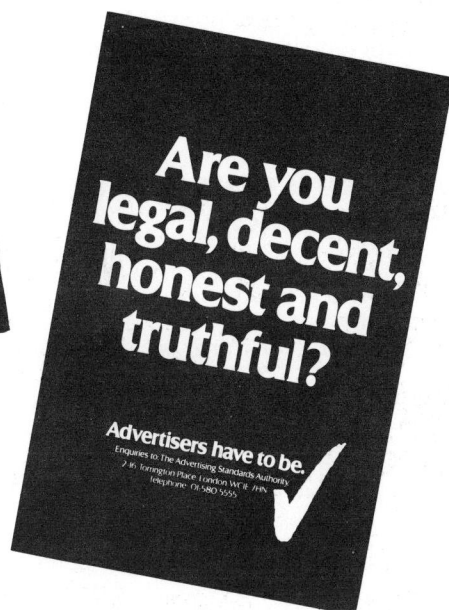

If an advertisement is wrong we're here to put it right.

The Advertising Standards Authority. ✓

Brook House, 2 Torrington Place London WC1E 7HN

Are you legal, decent, honest and truthful?

Advertisers have to be. ✓
Enquiries to The Advertising Standards Authority
2-16 Torrington Place London WC1E 7HN
Telephone 01-580 5555

Making Sense of it All

66 Eat your crusts. They'll make your hair curl! 99

How can you make sense of all the messages which you receive about health, especially when the messages often seem to conflict? Yesterday the advice was 'if you want to slim, avoid carbohydrates – cut out potatoes'. Today it's 'potatoes are a valuable source of fibre'. How do you know which piece of information to accept and which to ignore?

The following questions might help you to decide.

Who is giving the information?

We get information about health issues from a wide range of sources, including parents, friends, TV and doctors. Where does most of your information come from?

Working with 2 or 3 others, choose one of the issues from the box in the margin. Write down your issue in the centre of a large sheet of paper. Around it, jot down all the people that may have given you advice or information on this subject, over the years. Think back to when you were very young, to when you were at primary school, to when you were 13. Use these times in your life to pin-point as many sources of information as you can.

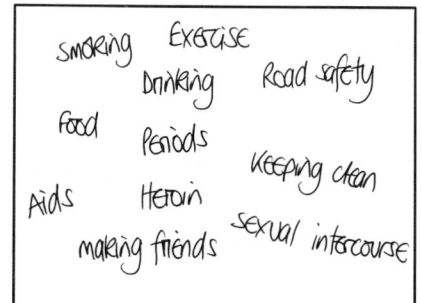

Underline the sources which you consider to be most reliable. If possible, compare your group's results with another's. Are your results similar, or do they vary depending on the issue in question?

If you were looking for advice, would you turn to the same people or sources now, as when you were younger? Discuss your reasons for underlining certain sources as reliable. Perhaps you consider these sources well informed. Are they qualified to give this information?

Sometimes we pick up information from surveys or research reported in newspapers, magazines or on TV. We may need to look long and hard to discover who is supplying the information. Who has funded the research and why?

> smoking Exercise
> Drinking Road safety
> food Periods
>   keeping clean
> Aids Heroin
>   sexual intercourse
> making friends

Why are you being given the information?

Is it to sell a product?

Is it to encourage you to act in a certain way?

Is it because the other person wants to seem knowledgeable? Countless 'myths' and stories are passed on from one person to another, often because the story-teller wants to seem as if they know it all . . . or have done it all.

66 Don't you know that? 99   *66 Haven't you ever done it? 99*

What information is being left out?

If the information is being given in order to promote a product, it is unlikely that any risks or dangers will be pointed out!

It is more likely that products will be glamorized.

If information is presented as a survey or research, check:

● Where it was conducted.
● Over how long a period of time and/or how often.
● How many people were involved.
● Any words which might make you doubt the results (words like 'seems', 'in some cases', 'perhaps', 'may').

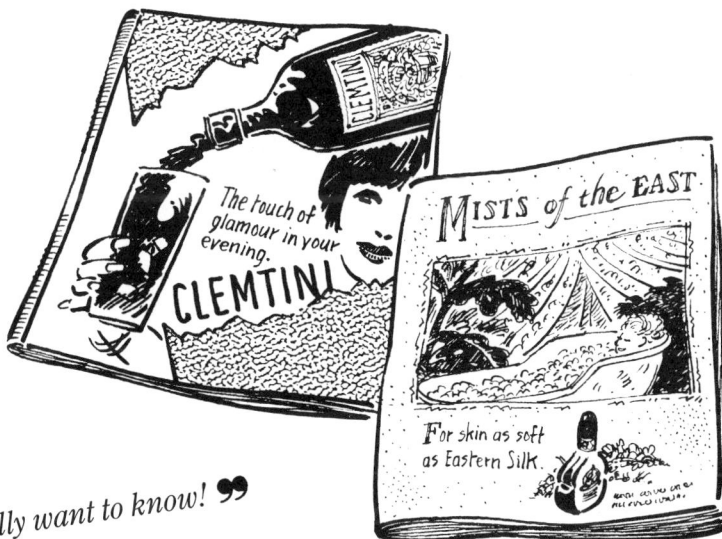

66 *Nobody ever tells us what we really want to know!* 99

Is the information accurate?

You could check this by asking a 'reliable' source – a person or an agency up-to-date with the most recent research and information. But remember, scientists are constantly coming up with new results, sometimes challenging past theories. At any point in time, all we can do is find out as much as we can, weigh up the facts and make decisions based on those facts.

Are you going to take any notice of the information given?

How much difference is this information really going to make to your life? Such information may influence us, but other factors also play a part in our decision to accept or reject it, such as whether it is practical, and whether it conflicts with our beliefs and our backgrounds. We look at this in more detail later on pages 20–23.

ACTIVITIES

» Collect a range of materials which give advice on health matters. You may find some useful information in supermarkets, chemists, at your doctor's or health centre, or in newspapers and magazines. Read through them, bearing all the above questions in mind. Which offer useful advice? Discuss your results in pairs.

» Identify a health message which you think it is important to give. Who would be the appropriate people to target? Design materials to put across that message, bearing in mind your target market.

Can we be Healthy all the Time

Have you ever had days when you've felt really down? Sometimes you may be physically ill with a headache, flu, or you may have an accident; other times you may feel depressed, fed up with everything and everyone. No matter who we are, surely nobody can feel completely healthy all the time?

ACTIVITIES

» Take a sheet of paper and draw a line on it to represent your life from birth (0) to your present age. Looking back over your life, have there been times when you have felt better than others? Perhaps certain events made you feel good or bad, for example, changing schools, changes in your family?

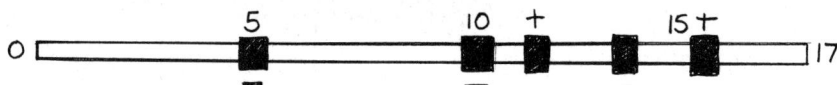

Mark a cross on the line for events which, in your opinion, affected how you felt (your health) in some way.

Next mark with a plus (+) sign those events which you think had a positive effect on your health, and with a minus (−) sign those which you think had a negative effect. Find somebody who you feel comfortable talking to. Choose two particular events on your line, which you would feel happy to discuss.

Each spend five minutes saying:

- What the events were.
- What effect each event had on your health.
- What, if anything, you learned from each event.

> It could be said that everything we experience is something which we can learn from.

» Role-playing in pairs as *A* and *B*: you have two minutes each to put your case.

A: We should avoid being hurt at all costs.

B: If I want to grow as a person, I need to take risks and maybe get hurt.

A: Childbirth should be a natural process, even if this is painful. It should involve as little medical interference as possible.

B: Medical interventions have made childbirth far safer. A pregnant woman should take advantage of the facilities and drugs available.

> 'Only people who avoid love can avoid grief. The point is to learn from it and remain vulnerable to love'   *John Brantner*

Choices

Throughout our lives we are faced with choices which may affect our health. As a small child many of these choices may be made for us, but as we get older most of us want and need to be independent and to make our own decisions.

Steps in decision-making

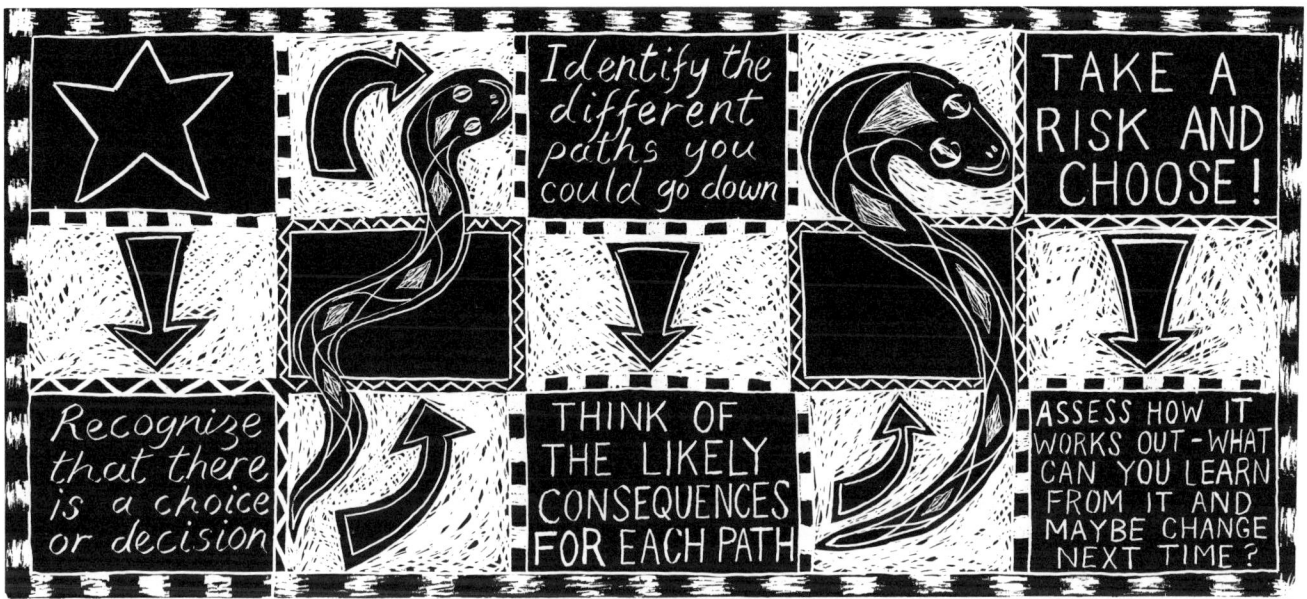

Often we *think* we know the choices we would make in a certain situation, but, when it occurs, we are surprised at how we react. For example, if you ask young teenagers if they would ever accept an illegal drug, most would say no. They may have an idea of a 'pusher' trying to sell them drugs at a school gate. In reality, the offer is far more likely to come from a friend. Their decision of whether to accept or not may not be so clear cut. It is likely to be influenced by a number of things, including how they are feeling at the time and who they are with.

For example, can you imagine these situations?

● At a party, towards the end of the evening, a friend of yours offers you some cannabis. Will you accept?
● During an evening out, the person you are with says that they have the house to themselves for the night. They want you to come back with them and maybe stay the night. Will you accept?

List all the things which are likely to affect your choice in these situations. (If you are stuck for ideas, there are some prompts at the bottom of the page.)

● Which are likely to be most important?
● What skills do you need to be able to cope?
● How much would your feelings and values affect your decision?

Prompts How you feel about the person you're with; whether they are male or female; your mood; parents' reactions; what you're supposed to be doing later; whether you've done it before; what you know about the likely consequences; whether you've been drinking; how sure you are of your own ideas and values.

19

Is it Easy to be Healthy?

Just suppose you decide that you want to be healthy and that you are going to make every possible healthy choice. You are going to give up smoking, limit your alcohol intake, eat the right food and take plenty of exercise. Is it going to be easy?

All the best intentions in the world are of no use, if the decisions are too hard to follow through. Many health choices are like New Year's resolutions: great in theory, but given up after a week! We all know people who are always planning to give up smoking or go on a diet, but they give up after a few days. Why is this?

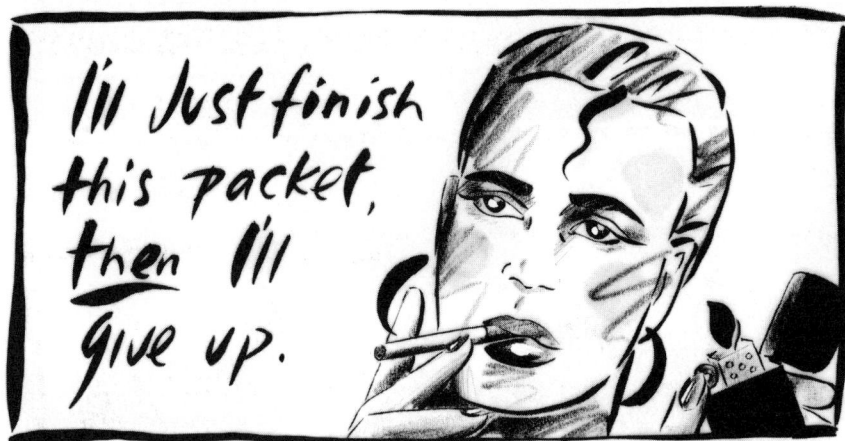

Why do you think people fail to carry through good intentions? Is it because they are:
- Lacking in will power?
- Easily swayed by others?
- Not really convinced?
- Lazy?
- Some other reason?

One part of the answer is that the decisions are often too difficult to persevere with. The personal cost of being healthy may be too great for the individual to pay. This is especially true if the costs are here and now and any possible benefits are somewhere in the distant future.

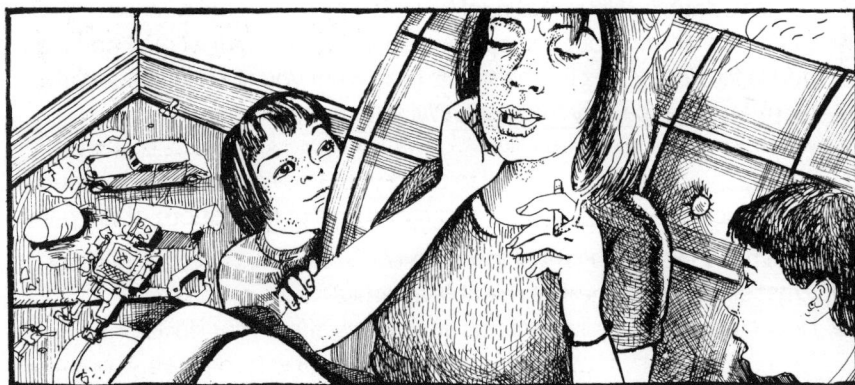

Some women, for example, say that smoking is their only pleasure. They use cigarettes to provide short breaks in their working day. Do you think this makes sense?

There are other reasons why the healthy choices may just be too difficult to follow. One such reason is the question of *availability*. For example:

- Is healthy food offered in the canteen?
- Are non-alcoholic drinks available in clubs/at parties?
- Is alternative transport available to discourage drinking and driving?
- Are sports centres and swimming pools in easy reach?

And another reason is *cost*. Anyone on a low income will have to think twice if the healthy option is more expensive. And in some cases it will be impossible for individuals to make the healthy choice, because they simply do not have enough money. Heating in winter, for example, may be essential to health but is a 'luxury' that some cannot afford.

ACTIVITIES

》 Think about how much your health is worth to you, in terms of 'personal cost'. What, if any, sacrifices would you be willing to make for the sake of your health?

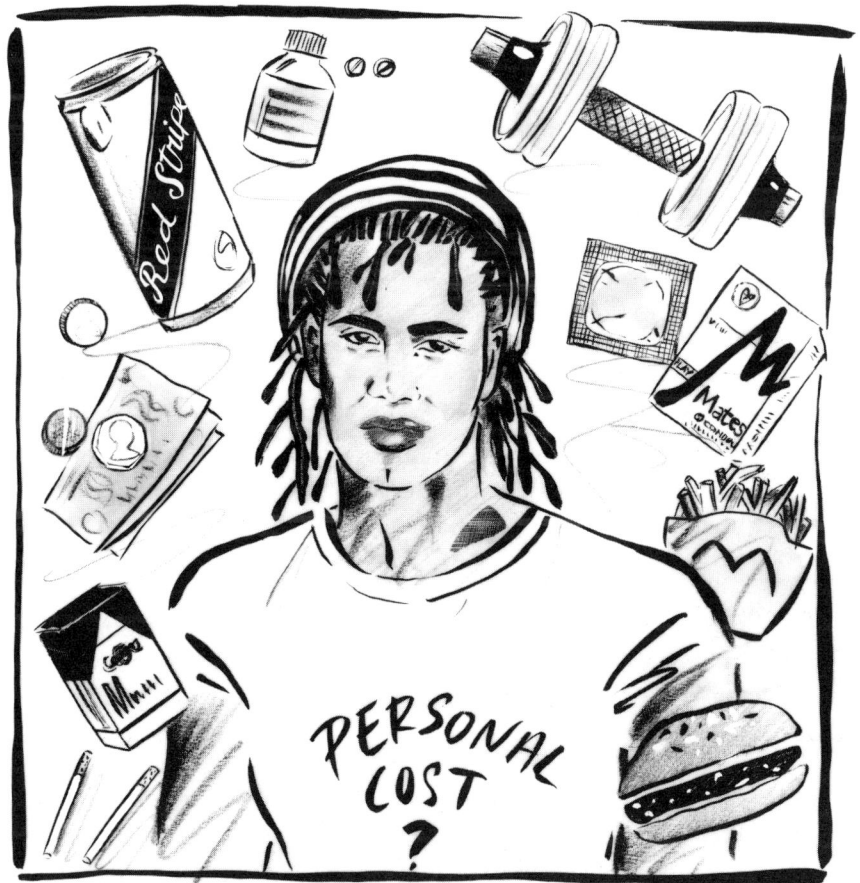

》 Write out a list of essentials for a young person choosing a healthy lifestyle and work out the cost for an average week. Discuss your findings and any possible savings that might be made on your original list.

》 Carry out a survey into the extent to which your school, college or local community promotes health by making healthy choices the easy choices. If you can suggest any improvements, you could send your ideas to your headteacher, principal or local MP. Your local paper might be prepared to carry an article or publish a letter about your findings.

*F*reedom of *C*hoice

Freedom of choice is thought to be very important in democratic countries but there are many areas of health where we have very little freedom as individuals.

How important, for example, do you think each of these is to health and well-being? Tick one of the boxes on the right and talk through your responses with another person, if possible.

	Very important	Quite important	Not important
Clean air, without fumes from factories or car exhaust.			
Safe roads and pedestrian or cycle paths.			
Clean water for drinking.			
Clean rivers and beaches for swimming.			
Areas of town and country set aside for recreation.			
Safe working environment.			
Conservation of energy supplies.			
Leisure facilities.			
Decent housing.			
Prevention of war.			
Protection of wildlife and natural habitats.			

When you have decided which are important to you, go back to the left-hand side of the statements and put a tick (√) if you think you have some control. Put a cross (X) if you think this area of health is outside your control.

When you have finished, think about the results and compare your answers with the views of others. Does it look as if there are important areas of health that are beyond the control of individuals? Can you think of others?

Most people expect that the Government will take care of these issues and that their health and safety is protected by the law. We expect that power stations will be run to high safety standards and that the water we drink will be completely safe. As individuals we elect a government and leave matters to them.

However, some people feel strongly that governments do not always concern themselves with health issues. Some may be so concerned with the economy, for example, that they leave health to chance. What do you think? Does the current Government do a good job of protecting our health?

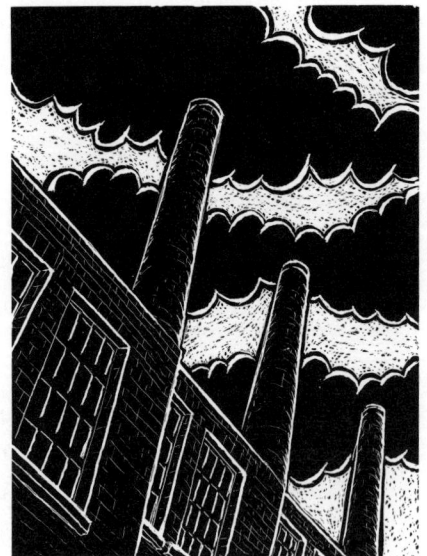

North Sea pollution sounds death knell for seals

The battle for our breathing space

Radioactive beef floats around the world

Children's playgrounds found to contain lead hazard

PESTICIDE POLICY ATTACKED

One way that individuals can make their feelings known and have some power, is by joining pressure groups that are concerned with health issues. There are dozens of these groups in Britain alone. They monitor what is actually happening to national health and campaign for government action where necessary. There are also local, volunteer groups that work to improve the environment – anything from cleaning up a river to planting trees.

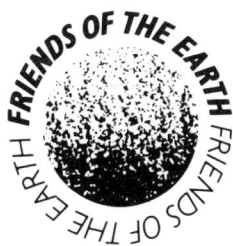

GREENPEACE

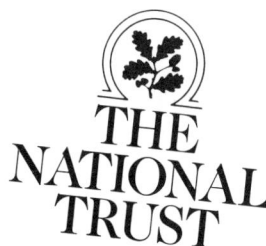

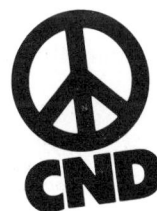

ACTIVITIES

» Find out about the work of pressure groups by writing to their national headquarters and/or by inviting in a local speaker.

» Join a local conservation group and get involved in practical work in your area.

» Use cameras to record the health problems of your local environment.

» Check back through local newspapers to find out about health problems in your community. How many of these are outside the control of individuals?

Health For All

One of the slogans of the World Health Organization is:

'Health for all by the year 2000'

This doesn't mean that everyone will be well all the time. But it means that everyone should have a *fair chance* of living a healthy life. And this should be true regardless of whether someone is male or female, black or white, living in a particular country or belonging to a particular social class.

Sadly, as we draw nearer the end of the century, this vision of health seems less and less likely to happen. Here in Britain, we are a very long way from having health for all our citizens. In 1980 the DHSS published a report entitled *Inequalities in Health*. (This became known as the Black Report, because it had been compiled under the chairmanship of Sir Douglas Black.) This report showed that manual workers and their families tend to die younger and have much worse health than professional men and women. More recent figures on inequalities in health were published by the Health Education Council in 1987 in *The Health Divide: Inequalities in Health in the 1980s* by M. Whitehead. The statistics on these two pages are for the early 1980s. They show up the differences in standards of health, according to social class.

Social class: according to the Registrar General's Scale		
Class I	professional	e.g. lawyer, doctor, accountant
Class II	intermediate	e.g. teacher, nurse, manager
Class III N	skilled non-manual	e.g. typist, shop assistant
Class III M	skilled manual	e.g. miner, bus-driver, cook
Class IV	partly skilled manual	e.g. farmworker, bus-conductor, packer
Class V	unskilled manual	e.g. cleaner, labourer

The bar charts below show the 'standardized mortality ratios' for the different class groups. In plain English this means that 100 equals the average death rate. Anything over 100 is worse than the average; anything less than 100 is better than average. So, the bar charts indicate a steep increase in death rates from Class I to Class V. Unskilled workers run at least twice the risk of death as professionals.

Mortality by social class, 1979–1983

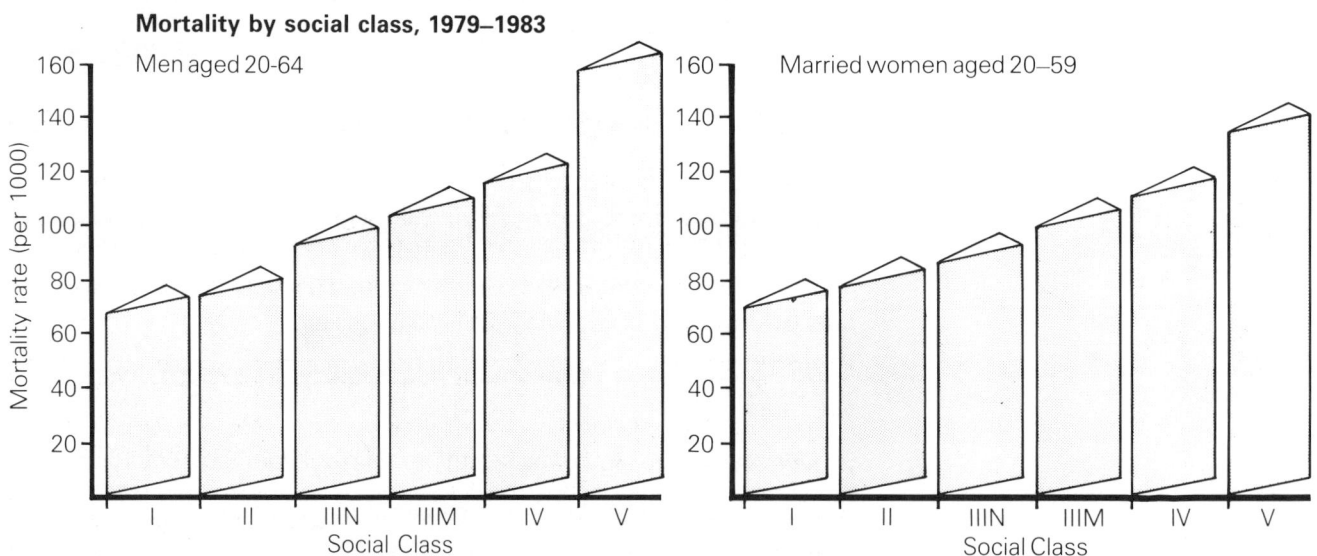

(Source: Office of Population and Census Studies)

But death rates are not the only evidence. The next bar charts below, show the percentage of the population reporting long-term illness. What does this tell us about:
● Differences between social class?
● Differences between men and women?

How does this chart compare with the ones shown opposite?

Percentage of the population reporting long-term illness, 1984

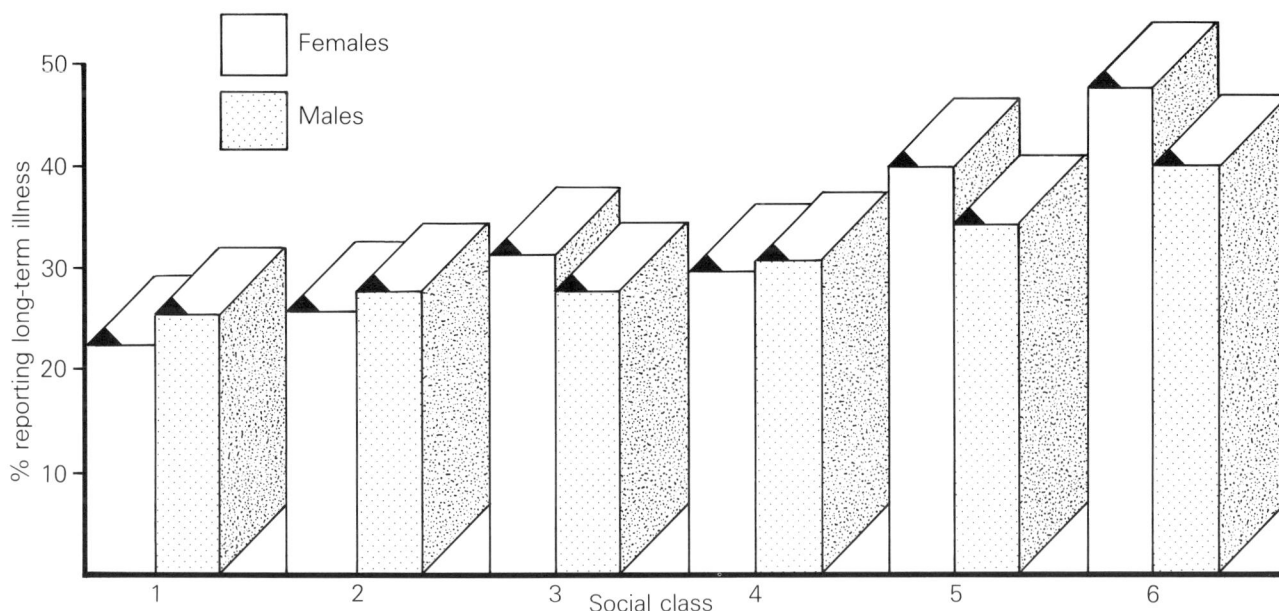

(Source: General Household Survey)

Almost all the statistics we could look at would tell the same story of inequalities in health between social classes.

The Black Report argued that such inequality was due to poverty, overcrowding and poor working conditions. The report recommended that:
● The emphasis should be on prevention rather than cure.
● Resources should go to the areas of greatest need.
● Society should make a better job of preventing poverty.

But since the report was published, unemployment and poverty have increased dramatically and there is no sign of a reduction in the inequalities of health to be found in Britain.

ACTIVITIES

» Social class is only one of the causes of inequalities in health. Other factors, such as where we live and the racial group we belong to, are also important. What factors do you think are important in your area? You could brainstorm your answers to this in a large, mixed group and then discuss the points you all find most important.

You could find out more about the effect of social class on health by sending for an inexpensive booklet called *The Unequal Health of the Nation* published by the TUC, Congress House, Great Russell Street, London, WC1B 3LS. The Black Report and *The Health Divide* have been published together in *Inequalities in Health* by Penguin Books, 1988.

The National Health Service

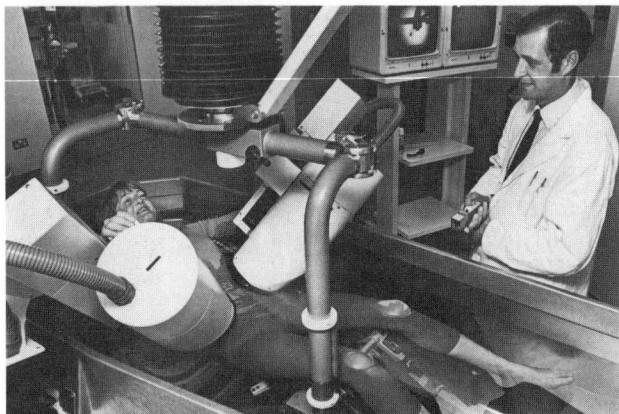

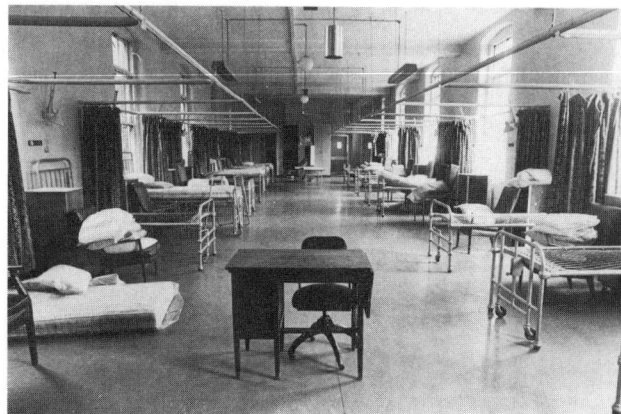

The NHS was set up in 1948 to provide free health care for rich and poor alike. It should have prevented some of the inequalities we looked at in the last section, but recently it has been severely criticized for failing in this. Although the NHS is the largest employer in Europe, it is ridiculed as the 'National *Sickness* Service' So, what really is the situation?

There are so many different arguments that it is best to begin with our own experience. What do you, your family or friends think about the comments shown here? Tick the column that matches your reaction to each comment.

	Agree	Disagree	Don't know
It's good not to have to pay for health services			
There is a clinic and hospital within easy reach of my home			
My doctor is readily available			
My doctor has time to talk through my problems			
The NHS waiting lists for hospital are exaggerated			
You get very good care in hospital			
The treatment in Britain is as good as anywhere in the world			
Private medicine doesn't really give you better care			

On the whole, the NHS *is* popular with its users. The fact that people no longer have to worry about paying for their doctor's services is a great achievement. The system works very cheaply compared with those in other countries. Provision for the elderly and disabled is better than in countries that rely on private insurance schemes. Many Americans envy our system because little provision is made for millions of their citizens.

However, it is also true that the NHS has many problems. There are long waiting lists and conditions are poor in many long-stay hospitals. The service is not equally efficient in all areas of the country. People complain that they are often pushed around, and that they are not consulted about their treatment.

There are many ways that the NHS could be improved. It would be better if the service was more 'user-friendly', so that people felt less frightened of hospitals and doctors. And the NHS also needs more resources in terms of staff, time and equipment. This requires more money and we all have to decide whether we are prepared for society to spend more on health services. Are we prepared to meet the cost of a modern, efficient health service?

Some people say that what we need are changes in the management and structure of the NHS. They think these would bring improvements without increased funding. What do you think?

▓ ACTIVITIES

》 Look through a selection of national and local newspapers and cut out all the articles about the National Health Service. What are the papers saying about the NHS? What are the main concerns? How could things be improved?

GPs vote to reject 'damaging' NHS changes

HOSPITAL WAIT LENGTHENS

Dangerous effects of health cuts

Nurses' fears of being downgraded to save money

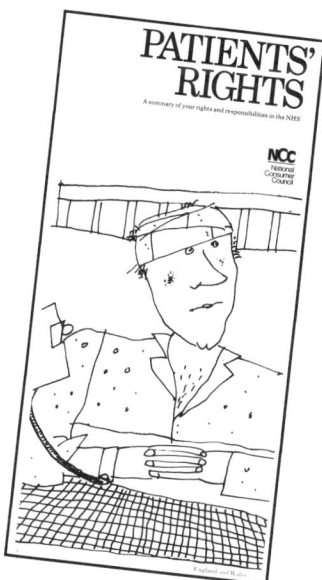

PATIENTS' RIGHTS
A summary of your rights and responsibilities in the NHS
NCC
National Consumer Council

》 You can find out more about your rights and responsibilities to the NHS, by reading this free *Patients' Rights* leaflet. Free copies can be obtained by writing to your local Community Health Council. You can find their address through your local library or in the telephone directory.

》 You could learn at first hand about services offered in your area in a number of ways:
● Invite in a range of speakers.
● Arrange visits or a placement in a local hospital.
● Carry out a survey of local provision.

Does the health service actually make people healthier?
I. Illich is a well-known writer, who argues that doctors and medicine just make us more dependent on services, but do not actually make us any healthier. He points to all the side-effects of drugs and the pain and suffering caused by doctors through the various forms of treatment. Another writer, T. McKeown, puts forward evidence that shows how little doctors have contributed to improvements in the nation's health. The main reasons we are all healthier are that we have better nutrition and clean water supplies – not because we go to the doctor!

》 Carry out a discussion (or even a formal debate) on the issue: 'Do doctors improve our health?'

Support Groups

After reading the last few sections you may be wondering whether opting for a healthy lifestyle is really too much trouble. Not only are some of the decisions very difficult to follow, but some are beyond your control. And the NHS isn't necessarily going to help much with any problems you may have. So where can you turn for help and support?

If you have a health problem it is obviously important to consult your doctor, but you may also be able to get help from a local support group. Sometimes called 'self-help', this depends on individuals meeting together to support one another.

Some of the ways they can help are shown here, but every group is different, depending on the needs of its members.

Support groups can provide:

● Advice.
● Information.
● Acceptance.
● The opportunity to meet people.
● The chance to talk with someone who 'understands'.
● A feeling of belonging to a group.
● Motivation to keep going.
● Support to bring about personal change.
● Support in changing social attitudes.
● Support in changing local provision laws, etc.

Some people feel that to turn to such a group amounts to admitting personal failure. Others think that in some way they would be letting down their family or friends.

What do you think? Is it fair to expect people always to be able to cope with their problems? Might it not even be a sign of strength for someone to 'take the plunge' and seek help from others with similar experience?

Supposing you did want to contact a support group – how would you go about it?

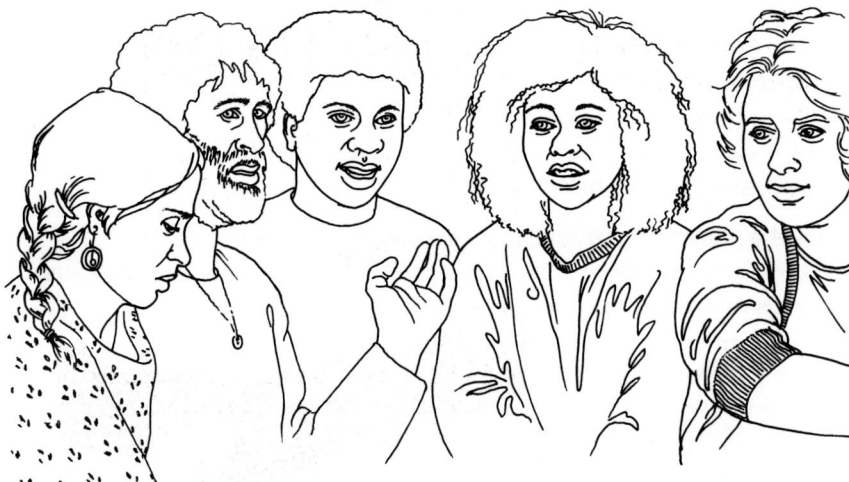

You could contact your local Social Services Department, Council for Voluntary Service, Community Council or Community Health Council. Or you could look out for posters advertising local support groups in health centres and local information offices.

You could write to the
National Council for Voluntary
Organizations or you could contact the
National Association of Young
Person's Counselling and Advisory
Services at:

17–23 Albion Street
Leicester
LE1 6GD

This association provides
information on counselling groups
run for young people throughout
the country.

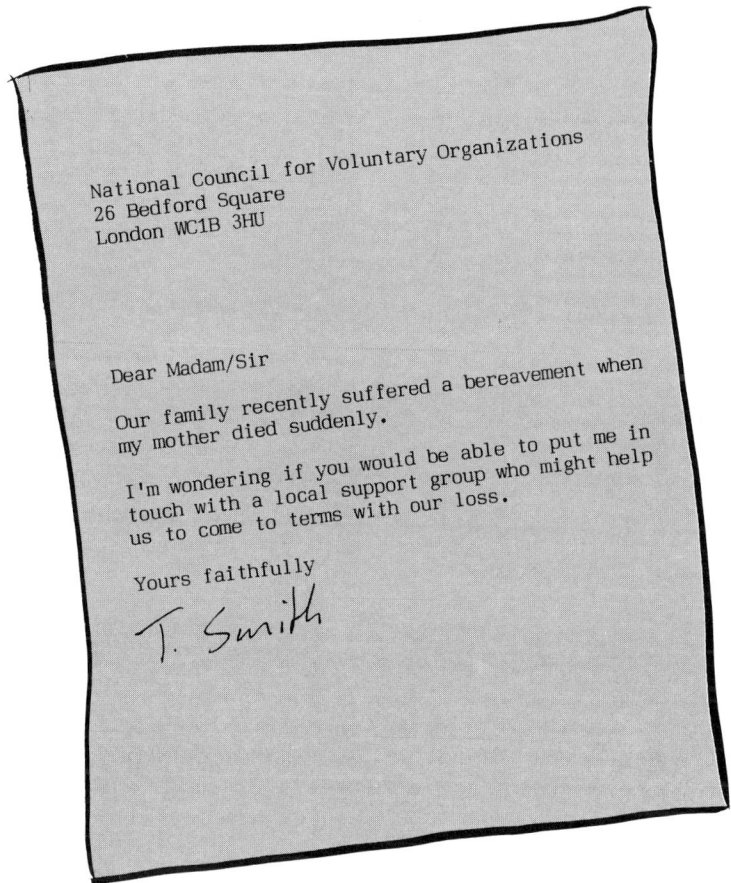

National Council for Voluntary Organizations
26 Bedford Square
London WC1B 3HU

Dear Madam/Sir

Our family recently suffered a bereavement when
my mother died suddenly.

I'm wondering if you would be able to put me in
touch with a local support group who might help
us to come to terms with our loss.

Yours faithfully

T. Smith

As you can see, there are a very wide range of organizations helping with
everything from losing weight to coming to terms with sexual
preferences. It's hard to think of an issue which is not covered by a group
but, even so, many people find that they have needs which are not catered
for. Sometimes it is then possible to start up your own group.

If you are interested in
starting a group or even
finding out more about
how groups work, you
could write for a copy of
*Self-Help Groups,
Getting Started, Keeping
Going* shown here. It is
available from:

Self Help Groups Project
20 Pelham Road
Notthingham
NG5 1AP

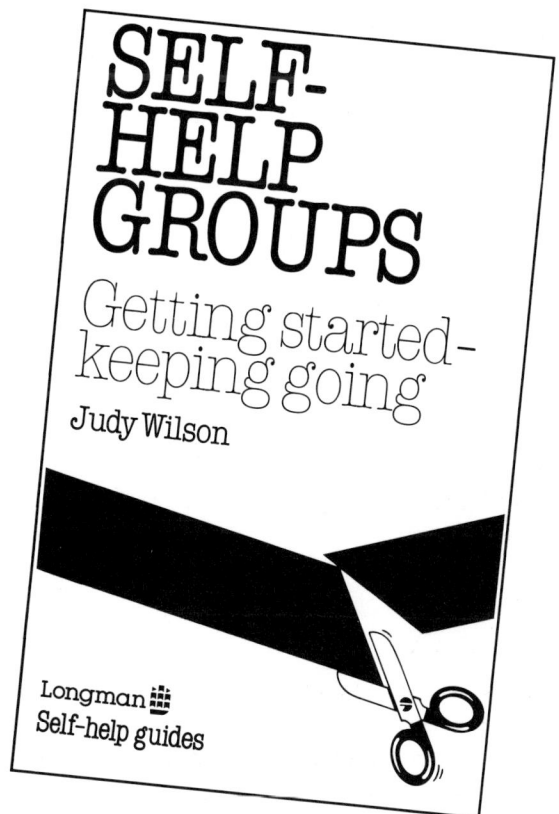

SELF-
HELP
GROUPS

Getting started –
keeping going

Judy Wilson

Longman
Self-help guides